DIY Oral Thrush Natural Home Remedies

The Effective Step by Step Guide to Permanently End Oral Thrush

Kantung Kim

Dedication

This book is dedicated to all who earnestly desire to cure their oral thrush.

Table of Contents

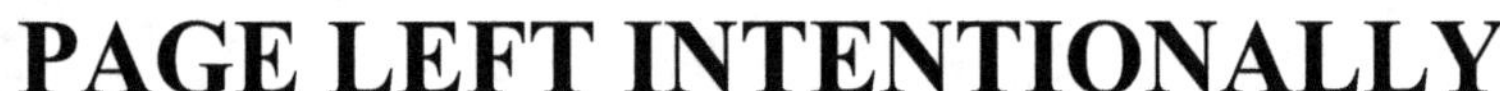

PAGE LEFT INTENTIONALLY

Introduction

Oral thrush which is also referred to as oral candidiasis is a yeast infection which occurs in the mouth and caused by a form of yeast in the mouth, caused by a kind of fungus which is called Candidiasis. The infection isn't contagious, meaning it cannot end up being passed to other people.

Oral thrush is a surface infection of the mucous membrane characterized by white adherent patches of pseudomycelium which frequently comprises of sores, fissures, lesions, and ulcers in the mouth which could either be acute or chronic.

It is accompanied with chronic illness and antibiotic therapy and is known to affect primarily elderly patients and small children. It is also common in severe HIV/AIDS infections.

Adaptable pathogens especially various Candida species residing in the human buccal cavity are the most common causes of oral thrush. These include C. parapsilosis, C. albicans, C. tropicalis, and other species of Candida.

They live as normal commensals when seen in these places but can cause infections when there is a change in their environmental conditions.

Candida species can also be quarantined in good quantity from the mouth of both healthy individuals who have no clinical evidence of Candida infection and persons who show clinical evidence of some previous identified oral infections.

When occurring in the mouth, the location of Candida colonization can alter between individuals and in the same individual from day to day. Other forms of fungi may be faced in oral thrush infection including Cryptococcus neoformans and Aspergillus sp.

Chapter 1

Oral Thrush

What Is Thrush?

Thrush occurs when the fungus Candidiasis rapidly grows on the mucus membranes of the mouth. It was originally described in 1838 by pediatrician Francois Veilleux. Candida originates normally in the mouth region, on the skin, in the mouth area and elsewhere, but bacteria and other inhabitants of a person's body generally keep fungal development in balance.

However, if the total amount of these habitually harmless organisms is changed, Candida can multiply, leading to fungal overgrowth and many medical problems, including oral thrush.

Symptoms of Oral Thrush

The most common symptoms of thrush are the appearance of white lesions in the inner cheeks. on your tongue and sometimes, the tonsils, the roof of the mouth, and gums. Other signs and symptoms of thrush includes:

1. Pain when attempting to swallow or having a difficult time swallowing

2. A burning, painful sensation of the tongue

3. A feeling of food sticking in the mid-chest or in your throat

4. Cracks at the corners of the mouth (i.e., angular cheilitis).

5. Soreness and redness on the inner part of the mouth.

6. Sore, white appearing patches (plaques) in the mouth that can be wiped.

7. A repulsive taste in the mouth which can either be a salty or bitter taste.

8. Fever (if the illness grows beyond your esophagus). Newborns with oral thrush usually become indicative in the first few weeks. There may be an appearance of white lesions in their mouths, experience hard time feeding or become unnecessarily cranky and irritable. Mothers whose breasts are infected with Candida may experience signs and symptoms such as:

1. Shiny skin on the areola

2. Unusual stabbing pains which makes you feel as though the breast is been pierced.

3. Red or tender nipples.

4. Discomfort when breastfeeding or having painful nipple between feedings.

Who Is Likely to Get Infected?

Infection is common in infants and toddlers whose immune systems aren't so strong. Nursing babies with thrush can pass the infection to their nursing mothers. You are also more likely to be affected by thrush if you:

1.Have a weak immune system

2. Smoke

3. Use dentures

4. Are an elderly person

5. Use antibiotics, birth control pills or corticosteroids.

Chapter 2

Causes of Oral Thrush

Oral thrush and various other Candida infections may appear when the disease fighting capability is compromised or suppressed by medications or when antibiotics modifies the normal balance of microorganisms in the body.

The oral thrush infections occur due to the rise of Candida albicans fungi that naturally appears within the mouth. This fungi rise may be caused by any of the following listed below:

1. A primary health issue such as HIV or cancer

2. Weakness of the immune system

3. The use of corticosteroid

4. Smoking

5. Mouth Injury

6. The use of specific medications to the reduce the quantity of saliva the mouth produces. You may have come across the word "Corticosteroids being used several times in this book" and may be wondering what it means or what it is been used for.

We are briefly going to let you in on the uses of Corticosteroids.

Uses of Corticosteroids

They are used in reducing inflammation (swellings) and in the treatment of certain illness such as:

1. Asthma, a long-term health condition which causes the airways of the lungs to be inflamed and swollen

2. Arthritis, A health situation which causes swelling of the joints and bones.

3.   Ezcema, a prolonged medical condition, affecting the skin that tiggers dry, itchy and red skin.

4.   Some specific types of cancer.

Most times, asthma is treated using inhaled corticosteroids. It is used by breathing through the recommended inhaler giving it a direct passage into the lungs. Even though, inhaled corticosteroids cause lesser side effects than other methods of treatment, they can alter the levels of acid in the mouth, thereby causing grave damage to healthy bacteria and causing a discrepancy that makes oral thrush to grow again.

In addition, frequent or prolonged use of antibiotics can wipe out bacteria which are friendly to the body and responsible for keeping the yeast in check, thus resulting in thrush.

Oral Thrush Diagnosis

Oral thrush is often diagnosed simply by having a health care provider or a dentist examine the white lesions; usually a tiny sample is examined under a microscope. If thrush appears in teens or older children with no possible factors, it is recommended to see a health practitioner, as an underlying health illness such as diabetes may be lurking around.

Thrush that stays in the oesophagus can be dangerous. Once this is observed, the doctor may advice an endoscopic examination, a throat culture or an upper GI test, precisely a barium swallow.

Facts About Oral Thrush

Many people have a wrong misconception about thrush. It is important you get your facts rights so as not to misinterpret the signs you notice in your health.

Oral thrush is a condition where the fungus causing thrush, Candida albicans amass on the lining of the mouth. Candida is a normal organism in your mouth, but it can become thick causing a painful symptom.

Anyone can be affected by oral thrush, however, its most common in newborn babies and the elderly as well as people with weak immune systems.

Overall, oral thrush is usually a minor problem if one is healthy, but when a person has a weakened immune system, then symptoms of oral thrush may be more severe or difficult to control.

Risk Factors

You are at higher risk of developing oral thrush if

1. You use dentures which are not properly fitted or cleaned regularly

2. You have high blood sugar levels in yor body

3. You are diabetic

4. You frequently use atibiotics medicine in combating infections

5. You have a deficiency in iron or suffer from Vitamin B deficiency.

Chapter 3

Treatment and Management of Oral

Thrush

The use of antifungal and maintaining a good oral hygiene is the best treatment for less severe oral thrush. In severe cases, medication can be recommended by your physician.

Treatment centers on Candida species. It must be targeted to the degree of the involvement and level of immunosuppression of the individual. Generally, antifungal agents are the suggested treatment. These antifungal agents treat infections by changing the DNA or RNA metabolism or causing intracellular growth of peroxide in the fungal cells.

For sufferers with a mild exhibition or having their first display of the health condition, topical treatment is the therapy recommended. One of such treatment is taking clotrimazole troches 10 mg orally five times a day.

Another option is using nystatin oral suspension (100,000 {units/mL), taking 5 mL orally four times daily. In the right conditions, another option is miconazole oral gel.

For moderate to serious illness, 200 mg of fluconazole should be taken orally once a day and then, 100 mg taken orally once daily for 7 to 14 days. This is considered safe for a breastfeeding mother.

In addition, a single dose of oral fluconazole 150 mg has proven to work in patients with advanced cancer, hence helping to reduce burden of pills.

Additionally, patients are to receive counseling on ways to decrease immunosuppressing challenges such as smoking, diabetes and malnutrition.

We have effectively discussed ways in which oral thrush can be successfully treated by taking antifungal medicines. You can find antifungal treatments available in these forms.

1. Lozenges

2.Creams

3.Tablets

4. Rinses (These are beneficial to people with dry mouth and find it difficult to swallow the antifungal tablets.)

Ensure you change or reduce the dosage of the antibiotics medicine or corticosteroids you are using if you observe that they cause you oral thrush.

Note: There are some antifungal medicines that should be avoided by a pregnant or breastfeeding woman. Ensure you get medical advice from your pharmacist or general practitioner before commencing the use of any antifungal medicines.

Possible Side Effects of Antifungal Medicines

The possible effects of using antifungal medicines are:

1. Headache

2. Stomach upset

3. Nausea

4. Indigestion

5. Diarrhea

If you are one of those that uses dentures, apply antifungal cream to the affected part of the mouth and to the lower part of your dentures. Also, using antifungal lozenges have proved to be effective.

If the original cause of your oral thrush cannot be treated, then, you may have to continue using antifungal medicine for a long period of time.

How to Prevent Thrush

Observing simple lifestyle changes can help to prevent thrush.

1. By all means, quit smoking and limit your consumption of alcohol.

2. Treat any other yeast infections you have as soon as possible.

3. Reduce your consumption of processed sugars.

4. Practice good oral hygiene and pay your dentist a visit regularly.

5. Use probiotics (from supplements or yogurt) when you take antibiotics.

6. Maintain a healthy and balanced diet.

7. Drink adequate water to keep your mouth moist.

8. If you are into dentures, make sure they are fitted.

9. Brush your mouth and floss regularly.

Chapter 4

Natural Treatment / Home Remedies for Curing Oral Thrush

Oral Thrush, called Oropharyngeal Candidiasis scientifically, is a medical ailment where your tongue or the internal side of the mouth area is contaminated by a kind of fungus known as CANDIDIASIS.

Now, let's dive into the various natural treatment that can be used in curing this infection without paying your doctor a visit.

1.**Salt.**

Salt is viewed as the best top home cures for treating oral thrush since it assists in destroying the fungus habitation. Also, when an infection occurs, using salt can decrease the symptoms of thrush and be a fast cure.

Method

A. You should mix ½ to 1 teaspoon of salt with a cup of warm water. With this solution, gargle and repeat the process until the symptoms observed are completely reduced and you feel more comfortable.

B. Apply some salt on the your tongue with your fingers, rub it in gently for a few seconds and then rinse your mouth with lukewarm water. This process should be repeated twice daily for a number of days.

2.Garlic

Even though some do not like the smell or taste of garlic, it is the best-known home cure for oral thrush because of its anti-fungal competence. Its capability helps to destroy yeast and bacteria present in the mouth and helps to boost the immune system.

Method

A. Eat two to three garlic cloves daily to protect yourself against infection. You can use the garlic that have been concentrated into capsules or tablets if you find it irritable to take fresh garlic, but this should be used only under your doctor's medical advice.

Garlic is also recognized to be exceptionally effective for diseases associated with oral health.

3.Yogurt

Do you know that probiotic yogurt is considered a harboring energetic form of lactobacilli which is considered very effective in treating oral thrush naturally? In addition, you are to use the unsweetened or plain yogurt to get the best cure for oral thrush.

Method

A. Take two to three cups of yogurt daily for a number of times in a week.

B. Wash your hands, apply a bit of yogurt to your tongue and the innermost part of the mouth with your finger and allow it stay for five to ten minutes. Once done, wash your mouth with warm water. This should be repeated daily for some number of days.

4.Cinnamon

Cinnamon is also good for its anti-fungal capability as well as its anti-parasitic capacity and effectively used for the treatment of Candida Albicans (Candidiasis).

For the effective use of cinnamon for oral thrush, A. Ensure you take one to two cups of cinnamon tea every day. Firstly, boil half teaspoon of cinnamon with one and half cups of clean water for five minutes. Once boiled, filter and drink your mixture with lemon or without lemon juice based on what you prefer. B. Pour in a few drops of cinnamon to a tablespoon of essential olive oil or other preferred product. Apply the solution directly to your thrush and allow to stay there for five to ten minutes, wash your mouth after this. This should

be repeated every day for a number of days.

5.CoconutOil

This is another useful and readily available cure for oral

thrush. It is extremely effective in removing the fungi and

relieving you of any unpleasant symptoms.

Method

A. Apply coconut oil directly to your thrush with a cotton

cloth. Repeat this process for a number of times per day for

six   to   seven   days.

B. Practice oil pulling every day on an empty stomach

using one tablespoon of coconut oil. Add a tablespoon of

coconut oil into your mouth, move the liquid in a circular

movement within the mouth for close to ten minutes, spit

out after this. Wash the mouth with tepid to warm water

and start your normal brushing of the teeth. Observing this

procedure everyday will guarantee you a good and hygienic oral health.

6.Baking Soda

This is one of the cheapest home cures for treating oral thrush and till date, still extraordinarily effective. It has the potency to crush the fungi that causes oral thrush. According to Brazilian Oral Analysis in 2009, it was broadcasted that 5% of sodium bicarbonate is extremely effective concerning treating oral thrush. Baking soda helps to balance the level of acid in your mouth. For the effective use of baking soda in the home, A. Add enough drinking water to one to two teaspoon of baking soda to form a paste. After this, use a piece of cotton fabric to apply the paste directly to the affected part.

Keep the paste in for some minutes and then rinse off with warm water. This should be repeated two to three times daily for several days.

B. Add ½ teaspoon of baking soda to a cup of water and wash the mouth area with it. Do this two times daily till the infection goes away.

7.AppleCiderVinegar

This provides enzymes that helps to combat the candida fungi and for this sole reason, it is dubbed as another top organic cure for treating oral thrush.

Vinegar will help to restore the pH level to its balance for it to control the further development of the fungus. Also, vinegar is known for its great influence on a person's immune system.

Method:

A. Mix two teaspoon of vinegar and half teaspoon of salt into a cup of lukewarm water. Wash the mouth area with this blend a couple of times each day till you notice signs of improvement.

B. Dilute two tablespoon of raw apple cider vinegar with

some raw honey into a cup of warmwater. This should be taken two times a day.

8.BlackWalnut

Black walnut is well-known for its richness in tannin containing strong anti-fungal and strong astringent competence.

If you are not comfortable eating this fruit, we have black walnut capsules and extracts to make using it more palatable.

9.Cranberry

This is almost like black walnut for its "arbutin", a compound accountable for getting rid of the Candida Albicans and recognized as a great natural cure for oral thrush.

For its effective use in the house,

A. Take cranberry tablets on a daily basis based on

directions. If you are to use this for children, using fresh cranberry is more suitable.

B. Take unsweetened and fresh cranberry juice for at least two times each day. Do this for two to three weeks until the fungus is removed.

10.Olive   Leaf

Olive Leaf is one of the most powerful & most effective home cures for the treatment of oral thrush because of its strong anti-fungi capability. Furthermore, the component, "oleuropein" plays a significant role as a strong for your immune   system.

For   effective   home   use   of   olive   leaf,

A. Take 250 to 500 mg of olive leaf (extracted) three times daily.

B. Also, there are olive leaf tea which can be made by simply soaking the olive leaf in boiling water for approximately 15 minutes. Take two to three cups of this mix each day. Please note that, once you see a change, you should continue to drink one to two cups every day to prevent the re-emergence of candida fungus.

In addition to all that has been discussed above, here are extra tips for you to adhere to. Ignoring this whilst observing the home remedies may be a waste of time on your part.

A. Your toothbush should be changed regularly.

B. Make use of cotton cloth or better still, a scraper for the tongue to clean the tongue regularly.

C. Avoid smoking if the thrush gets worse.

D. For persons with dentures, ensure you do not wear to sleep. Keep your dentures in a denture cleaning liquid overnight. Always use clean toothbrush and water for cleaning your denture.

E. Limit your consumption of sugar to prevent further growth of fungus.

F. Whilst on this infection, take only food which will be easy to chew and swallow.

G. Brush your teeth twice daily, floss once and avoid sharing toothbrush.

H. Diabetic persons should monitor their sugar level to prevent infection.

I. See your dentist on a regualr basis exspecially persons with diabetes and those using dentures.

J. Consume ice water to ease any discomfort you have.

ExtraTips:

Change   toothbrush   regularly For folks using dentures, usually do not wear to sleep and retain in denture cleaning liquid overnight. Make use of clean toothbrush and drinking water for denture cleaning. Diabetic patient needs to monitor their glucose level to avoid   further   infection.

Eat food simple to chew and easy to swallow.

Visit your dentists regularly, most especially, individuals who have dentures and diabetes.

Chapter 5

Foods to Avoid

The candida diet, being a strict diet eradicates alcohol, gluten, and some dairy products. Candida diet advocates believe these foods promote candida overgrowth.

Doing away with these foods has not been established to be helpful against candida infections. However, studies proposed that, the excessive intake of sugar may worsen infections in mice with a deteriorated immune system (21Trusted Source).

I have listed some foods to avoid stopping the occurrence of oral thrush:

1. Certain meats such as farm-raises fish and deli meats.

2. High-sugar fruits like dates, bananas, mango, grapes and raisins.

3. Refined fats and oils such as soybean, sunflower oil, margarine, and Canola oil.

4. Grains containing gluten like barley, wheat, spelt and rye.

5. Certain dairy products such as cream, milk, and cheese.

6. Condiments such as soy sauce, mayonnaise, ketchup, BBQ sauce, white vinegar, and horseradish.

7. Alcohol, caffeine, and sugary beverages such as energy drinks, wine or spirits, caffeinated teas, soda, beer, coffee, fruit juice.

8. Nuts and seeds higher in mold like pecans, cashews, pistachios, and peanuts.

9. Sugar and artificial sweeteners such as table sugar, corn syrup, agave, aspartame, cane sugar, honey, molasses and maple syrup.

10. Additives such as nitrates or sulfates.

In addition, ensure you avoid high sugar foods, processed foods, fats and oils, additives, caffeinated drinks as well as alcoholic drinks.

Foods to Eat

1. High-quality protein foods such as eggs, turkey, chicken, salmon, and sardines (go for organic, pasture-raised and wild-caught varieties).

2. Non-caffeinated beverages like homemade almond milk. Filtered water, herbal teas, coconut milk (without additives), chicory coffee, and water infused with lime or lemon.

3. Low-sugar fruits like berries (eaten in small amounts), limes, lemon.

4. Herbs and spices such as paprika, ginger, turmeric, cinnamon, black pepper, dill, salt, garlic, oregano, rosemary, and thyme.

5. Non-starchy vegetables like tomatoes, broccoli, eggplant, spinach, asparagus, cabbage, brussels sprouts, kale, cucumber, celery, onion, zucchini, and rutabaga (best eaten steamed or raw).

6. Healthy fats such as flax oil, avocado, sesame oil, olives, unrefined coconut oil, and extra-virgin olive oil.

7. Gluten-free grains, e.g., oat bran, buckwheat, millet, and quinoa.

8. Certain dairy products such as plain yogurt, butter organic kefir or ghee.

9. Nuts and seeds low in mold like flaxseed, sunflower seeds, coconut or almonds.

10. No-sugar sweeteners such as erythritol, stevia, and xylitol.

Furthermore, probiotic supplements may help relieve inflammation, eradicate harmful organisms and decrease the occurrence of candida and infection symptoms (18Trusted Source, 19Trusted Source, 20Trusted Source).

Chapter 6

Conclusion

Oral candidiasis is linked with having systemic diseases and intake of medication, particularly with those medications can cause xerostomia. As the number of systemic diseases and medications increases, the danger of developing oral candidiasis may also increase.

Oral thrush, if effectively treated can be cured, never to resurface again. Again, this doesn't happen by luck, it takes due diligence on your part.

Adhere strictly to the diet recommended by your doctor, avoid foods and beverages that easily trigger oral thrush and you will be just fine.

And above all, regular visit to your doctor is very important.

To your health.

Disclaimer

Although, the author have made every effort to ensure that the information in this book was correct at press time, the author do not assume and hereby disclaim any liability to any part for any loss, damage, or disruption caused by errors or omissions, whether such errors or omissions result from negligence, accident, or any other cause.

Did you enjoy reading this book, please consider leaving a

review to help us serve you better

Thank You.

About The Author

Kantung Kim is a father, husband and a writer. He loves reading, writing and hiking.

www.ingramcontent.com/pod-product-compliance
Lightning Source LLC
Chambersburg PA
CBHW050749250726
48662CB00005B/2114

* 9 7 9 8 6 2 5 6 6 0 9 0 7 *